FIRST,
WEAR A
FACE MASK

RODALE

FIRST, WEAR A FACE MASK

A DOCTOR'S GUIDE TO REDUCING RISK OF INFECTION DURING THE PANDEMIC AND BEYOND

DR. PHILIP M. TIERNO, JR.

No book can replace the diagnostic expertise and medical advice of a trusted physician. Please be certain to consult with your doctor before making any decisions that affect your health, particularly if you suffer from any medical condition or have any symptom that may require treatment.

Copyright © 2020 by Philip M. Tierno, Jr., PhD

Published in the United States by Rodale Books, an imprint of Random House, a division of Penguin Random House LLC, New York.
rodalebooks.com

RODALE and the Plant colophon are registered trademarks of Penguin Random House LLC.

Library of Congress Cataloging-in-Publication Data
Names: Tierno, Philip M., author.
Title: First, Wear a Face Mask / Philip M. Tierno, Jr., PhD.
Description: New York : Rodale Books [2020] | Includes index.
Identifiers: LCCN 2020023955 (print) | LCCN 2020023956 (ebook) |
ISBN 9780593233030 (paperback) | ISBN 9780593233047 (epub)
Subjects: LCSH: COVID-19 (Disease) | COVID-19 (Disease)—Health aspects.
| COVID-19 (Disease)—Safety measures.
Classification: LCC RA644.C67 T54 2020 (print) | LCC RA644.C67 (ebook) |
DDC 616.2/414—dc23
LC record available at lccn.loc.gov/2020023955
LC ebook record available at lccn.loc.gov/2020023956

ISBN 978-0-593-23303-0
Ebook ISBN 978-0-593-23304-7

Printed in the United States of America

Book design by Meighan Cavanaugh
Cover design by Anna Bauer Carr
Cover art: ghrzuzudu/Shutterstock

10 9 8 7 6 5 4 3 2 1

First Edition

To all the brave healthcare workers, first responders, scientists, members of the military, and a myriad of others, especially service workers, who chose to work through the COVID-19 pandemic, many of whom paid the ultimate price. They sacrificed themselves and rose to the challenge, exceeding all expectations for the benefit of their fellow man.

CONTENTS

FIRST,
WEAR A
FACE MASK

AN OUNCE OF PREVENTION

F or the moment, let's take a step backward in order to fully assess what happened to us as individuals, as citizens, and as members of the global community during the spread of COVID-19. Simply put, the lives of every member of our human civilization on planet Earth were completely disrupted and changed by the lowest life-form on earth—an invisible germ!

The sheer enormity of that is a stark realization: a pandemic caused by a virus literally closed down America as well as the rest of the world. Nothing can better exemplify the interconnectedness of man and microbes than the COVID-19 pandemic. We humans are only part of the web of life on earth, and our well-being depends upon an intimate cooperation with the lowly germ! Even though the science of microbiology is little more than a century old, we have learned a lot about germs. We must use that body of knowledge to prevent catastrophic disruptions on earth like the one caused by the COVID-19 virus. To do that requires *all* of us (scientific and medical personnel as well as the public) to understand the dynamics at play so that we all follow the known basic protocols for fighting an infection, or for that matter, a pandemic.

While the story of the novel coronavirus COVID-19 is still unfolding as I'm writing this book, it is important to recognize that in a global economy of mass migration and frequent travel, there is no such thing as an isolated population group, and there is certainly no guarantee that a disease outbreak in that population won't go global in a couple of days.

From a public health perspective, the world's population is one big family. An outbreak in China concerns people in London, L.A., and New York City. Our past history indicates that it is easy to predict that infectious diseases, both old and new, will continue to emerge and challenge the world's established medical and scientific infrastructures from time to time. In order to meet that challenge we must educate all countries and their people about ways to prevent infection. Doing so would do more to enhance health, at a lower cost, than would any form of treatment. The new novel coronavirus has reemphasized the need for every person to understand the basic dynamics of infectious disease, to learn how we make each other sick and what we can do to protect our loved ones as well as ourselves.

This book will help you learn how we make each other sick and how to increase your chances of evading infection—which not only has obvious benefits to your personal well-being, but also breaks the chain of infection transmission. The COVID-19 virus had an unprecedented impact on the world. It caused a pandemic involving more than 200 countries and territories complete with a worldwide economic disaster, financial collapse, and adverse psychological manifestations for the masses. There clearly is a need to present information—in a concise, straightforward, and non-hyperbolic manner—on how we can understand and then mitigate any such infections in the future.

There is unfortunately a proliferation of false, contradictory, or simply overwhelming information on the Internet. Figuring out how to stay safe in this changed world by watching the news, searching on websites and social media, or listening to your friends can feel like drinking from a fire hose. As a microbiologist with forty-plus years' experience, I've set out to share the most important information about how infections spread and how you can stay safe from all manner of contagious diseases in a digestible, approachable, and even reassuring manner. If you want to get straight to the strategies, turn to page 41. I'll walk you through the most common scenarios you'll encounter in everyday life: commuting, traveling, cooking, and keeping your house, kids, and pets safe. But after you've grounded yourself in these important life skills, I encourage you to flip back to Part 1 and learn the larger context of how infections spread through populations. This will help you sift through what you hear on the news and from health authorities so that you can take your health into your own hands.

With this book, you can feel assured in arming yourself both against false information with a basic understanding of infectious diseases and against infection itself with best practices. As the old adage advises, "An ounce of prevention is worth a pound of cure."

PART 1

EVERYTHING YOU NEED TO KNOW ABOUT GERMS

1

WHAT'S A CORONAVIRUS?

You probably picked up this book because you're worried about COVID-19, so let's start there.

Coronaviruses are a worldwide group of RNA (ribonucleic acid, the genetic material of some viruses) viruses that were first identified in the 1960s. Bacterial and human cells have both RNA and DNA, but viruses have either one but not both, because they are more primitive cell types. They are the cause of about 15 to 30 percent of common colds, usually in the winter months. The primary symptoms produced are similar to another cold virus, rhinoviruses (which cause about 50 percent of common colds), and both are typified by an upper respiratory infection with a stuffy nose (loss of smell and taste are common), coughing (usually dry), varying fever, malaise, and fatigue.

Some adults carry the virus without fever. And most of these ordinary strains are treated with over-the-counter medications for the symptoms that they cause. The infection rarely spreads to the lower respiratory tract to cause pneumonia. That's more likely to occur in people who are older, or who have comorbidities like COPD, heart disease, diabetes, or are immunosuppressed.

Studies have shown that antibodies to the coronavirus appear in childhood and increase with age. It has also been shown that people can be *reinfected* in some cases after a period of about a year (that's why respiratory viruses continually cause colds in humans), although immunity usually lasts longer, and maybe even for life. Coronaviruses are also suspected of causing gastroenteritis, with the virus sometimes found in the stool. Animals also have infections caused by coronaviruses, but their viruses usually do not infect humans and, vice versa, human strains don't usually infect animals.

Sometimes, however, they do. An outbreak of a novel coronavirus that jumped from animals to humans, called SARS (severe acute respiratory syndrome), occurred in

South China in late 2002 and, by the time it waned in mid-2003, resulted in 8,000 cases in 29 countries, with more than 800 deaths (a case fatality rate of 10 percent). Clearly, we learned in that outbreak that animal coronaviruses can mutate and jump from animal species to humans. In fact, a perfect evolutionary melting pot occurred in the Chinese open-air animal market where people commingled with animals daily. These animals were slaughtered on the spot and then packaged and sold to people who used them in ritual ceremonies or for food delicacies.

Coronaviruses have the ability to exhibit a high frequency of mutation, and an especially high incidence of deletion mutations. They also undergo a high frequency of recombination during replication. This becomes a perfect prerequisite for a mutation that allows jumping species from animals to humans. It is believed that the SARS virus, for example, jumped from a bat to a civet cat to humans. In 2012 there was another coronavirus outbreak called MERS (Middle East respiratory syndrome). According to the CDC, health officials first reported the disease in Saudi Arabia in September 2012 but later identified that the actual first MERS case occurred in Jordan in April 2012. It then spread from the Middle East to Africa, Asia, and Europe. In May 2015 there was an outbreak of MERS in Korea, which was the largest outbreak recorded at that time. The MERS virus has a reservoir in camels and had the highest mortality rate, 35 percent.

Next comes the new coronavirus disease of 2019 (aka HCoV-19, COVID-19, nCoV-19, SARS-CoV-2). I will use the COVID-19 designation, which really refers to the disease caused by the virus, for convenience. This strain of virus is different from all others in that it causes more severe disease, especially in older adults, than the seasonal flu but less severe than SARS and MERS. This novel coronavirus likewise originated from animals and jumped from animal species to humans. It has been reported that in the open-air animal market in Wuhan, China, it likely spread from a bat (the COVID-19 virus is almost identical to a bat coronavirus), then likely to a pangolin (scaly anteater), and then to humans via a mutation that occurred during replication.

Several researchers have genetically traced the origin of the New York strains of the COVID-19 virus and found that it most resembled European strains. Hence the original virus started in Wuhan, China, traveled to Europe, and then finally a traveler from Europe brought it to New York. The West Coast received the Wuhan strain from passengers traveling from China to L.A. By 2020 it takes the prize of all previous coronavirus infections. It is spread by direct and indirect contact from one person to another via large aerosol droplets of greater than 5 microns (micrometers) in diameter as well as via airborne droplets (smaller droplets) less than 5 microns in size. The virus has also been reported to remain suspended in the air for at least 3 hours. Indirect spread occurs from contaminated surfaces being touched by hands and then those hands touching your nose, mouth, or eyes, which are the conduits of entry into your body. **That is why handwashing is the single most important thing you can do to protect yourself!**

In addition to the virus having been reported to remain in the air for about 3 hours, it is also able to live on a copper surface for 4 hours, cardboard for 24 hours, and on non-porous plastics and stainless steel for 3 days. The good thing is that soap and water can easily kill the virus because the virus has an outer envelope, which is rich in lipids. Most other common disinfectants will also kill this virus. (You can buy either sprays or wipes with a disinfectant claim on the label; when a product claims to be a disinfectant, that means the product destroys or inactivates both the bacteria and viruses noted on the label, whereas sanitizers only reduce the number of bacteria. Make sure you follow the package's directions about how long the spray needs to sit on the surface before being wiped away.)

Although the virus has been reported to live on some nonporous surfaces for up to 3 days, studies show that its infectivity diminishes over time on these surfaces. It is also important to understand that there have been early indications that individuals infected with COVID-19 may shed and transmit the virus when they are presymptomatic, symptomatic, or postsymptomatic. Several reports have confirmed that approximately 25 percent of people infected with the COVID-19 virus have no symptoms and don't know that they are infected. It has been reported that more virus is actually spread presymptomatically than when symptoms occur. On a good note, there have been studies from China that suggest that there is no transmission from mothers to their fetuses. In addition, the virus has not been found in samples of amniotic fluid or breast milk. Experts aren't sure about young children. If kids get the virus, they are generally not that sick (although there are exceptions). They apparently have mostly mild illness, but even children with mild cases can potentially spread the virus to other people, including the elderly. Of course, there are exceptions to every rule. Rarely, some children have been reported to get a potentially fatal hyperimmune inflammatory syndrome (a Kawasaki-like disease).

Most at risk for a serious infection are those individuals with comorbidities like high blood pressure, diabetes, or COPD, and the immunosuppressed. Also at high risk are obese individuals, smokers, vapers, and anyone older than 65. The novel COVID-19 virus is at least 3 to 4 times more contagious than the flu virus is.

2

HOW TO STOP AN EPIDEMIC

The definition of *epidemic* is "a widespread occurrence of an infectious disease in a community at a particular time." (Whenever an epidemic disease spreads across a large region or has spread globally it is referred to as a *pandemic*.) An epidemic can result in the healthcare system of a country becoming unable to handle such a large-scale crisis. Hence the goal is to *slow the spread* of disease over time.

You've seen the graphs representing the number of cases over time. In an epidemic, it looks like a *bell-shaped curve*, with a big spike of cases in a period of time. When we slow the spread of disease, we *flatten the curve*, allowing for the healthcare system to accommodate the sick, especially if critical care beds with ventilators are needed (as is the case with COVID-19). This is to prevent dealing with a large surge of cases over a short period of time that cannot be accommodated, and which might result in a larger number of deaths.

HOW DOES AN EPIDEMIC FINALLY END?

Generally speaking, an epidemic in a country can end when any *one* of the following four criteria are met:

1. **Everyone who can possibly get infected gets infected.** An extreme example of this is the so-called Spanish flu of 1918–19. That pandemic infected approximately one-fourth of the population of the U.S. and killed an estimated 675,000. Globally, roughly 500 million people were infected, with a death toll estimated at 20 to 50 million.

2. **The government finds everyone who is infected through rigorous testing for the germ** and then quarantines them to prevent further spread. They then

engage in tracing contacts by testing everyone who interacted with the infected person. If positive, they too would be quarantined. During an epidemic the government may also apply additional steps like "social distancing," "shelter in place," "stay at home," and even "self-quarantining," for a prescribed period in order to curb spread (see pages 51-52). Use of face masks (see page 49) is also recommended at this time to assist in curbing the spread. The cornerstone of the way forward before reopening a country is testing for *antibodies* to the germ to understand the level of population that has immunity, in addition to continuing testing for the virus. The people who have antibodies are generally able to safely return to work without fear, as they are protected from the virus. This process is how the SARS and Ebola outbreaks were eventually ended.

3. **A natural seasonal transmission via warm weather slows down the spread.** A good example of this is the yearly influenza that peters out with the advent of warmer weather, as do ordinary coronaviruses. (It is unknown if this is applicable to COVID-19 at the time of writing.)

4. **If there is an effective vaccine or drug treatment that would be able to prevent or treat the disease.** An example of this is the annual influenza vaccine, which helps to provide herd immunity to a population. *Herd immunity* results when a sufficiently high number of individuals (about 60 to 80 percent) are immune to the disease, whether through a vaccine or from recovering from the disease. It is hoped that as a result of an initial outbreak of an infectious disease in a population, a second or subsequent outbreak either won't occur or will be greatly reduced as a result of herd immunity.

CONTAINING AN EPIDEMIC: SOUTH KOREA

In the early stages of the COVID-19 outbreak, the worst-hit population outside of Mainland China was South Korea. But their response to the outbreak serves as a grand example to the world of their relative success in containing COVID-19 in their country. The key to their success was the timely implementation of government action to find everyone who was sick by massive testing, and then quarantining them, preventing further spread. They also implemented other very strict controls. The South Korean government tested more than a quarter of a million people in short order. They were able to test up to 20,000 people a day at more than 600 testing sites nationwide, including pop-up facilities and drive-through clinics.

By comparison, the United States had tested only a fraction of that at a similar point in time. Some states have actually copied the South Korean model of drive-throughs and pop-ups, but because access to testing woefully lagged behind in the United States, it was too late to have a success equal to South Korea's. The U.S. president had also defunded the very pandemic agency (National Security Council Directorate for Global Health Security and Biodefense) that would have helped to contain this threat and initially denied that the virus would become an epidemic in the U.S. That contrasted with the South Korean president, who took a backseat to the health professionals who called the shots. He took the outbreak quite seriously and allowed the medical and scientific professionals to run the response. As the South Korean minister of foreign affairs told reporters, "Openness and transparency build public trust and that leads to a very high level of civic awareness and voluntary cooperation that strengthens our collective effort to overcome this public health emergency."

FAILURE TO CONTAIN AN EPIDEMIC: ITALY

Italy was the first country outside of China to experience the wrath of COVID-19. While South Korea is a story of success, Italy is an example of failure, because they ignored professional warnings of experts. Many public health officials had sounded the alarm that Italy needed to take steps to use coronavirus testing to identify people with the disease, and then to quarantine those found with disease while also enforcing social distancing. As a result of not heeding the warnings, the curve was not flattened. The hospitals and medical personnel were overwhelmed. Because of that, those Italian physicians had to navigate difficult choices of prioritizing the life and death of patients, which was very reminiscent of catastrophic World War II wartime triaging.

TYPHOID MARY AND OTHER SUPER-SPREADERS

By definition, a super-spreader is an unusually contagious germ-infected individual who is more likely to infect someone than a typically infected individual. Whenever someone talks about the ability of a super-spreader to infect many people, Typhoid Mary comes to mind. Typhoid fever is a human disease caused by the bacterium *Salmonella typhi*. An Irish immigrant whose proper name was Mary Mallon worked as a cook in various New York City households under assumed names in the first years of the twentieth century (from 1901 to 1915). She had to use a series of false names because she made people sick wherever she worked. Although she herself had no symptoms and remained healthy, she carried the germ that caused typhoid fever and she transmitted it to her employers, their families, and their guests in the cakes, puddings, and other dishes she made as well as through the things she touched. At the time, there were no antibiotics available to treat her.

New York City health authorities eventually detained her in a hut on the grounds of an isolation hospital on North Brother Island in the East River. She sued for her release, which was granted after a few years on the condition that she work not as a cook but in laundry, where she was to handle only the dirty clothes. But the kitchen was her calling, and in 1915 she went back to work as a cook under a false name in, of all places, the kitchen of a maternity hospital. A fresh outbreak of typhoid fever followed, including two deaths. She was apprehended again and again quarantined on North Brother Island, with only her dog for company, until her death twenty-three years later. In all, Typhoid Mary infected more than fifty people with typhoid fever bacteria and was responsible for three deaths.

There have been several other outbreaks of disease spread by super-spreaders. Aside from COVID-19, the most recent was the SARS outbreak in 2002–2003. That outbreak originated in mid-November of 2002 in China's Guangdong province. There was also the highly contagious measles outbreak that occurred in 1989. This airborne virus even appeared in vaccinated populations. However, the most impressive outbreak involving super-spreaders is COVID-19. There's mounting evidence of super-spreading events, which were associated with both explosive growth early in the outbreak and sustained transmission in later stages.

There is a simple mathematical equation that relates to super-spreaders called R0 (R-naught):

$$R0 = \text{number of contacts} \times \text{shedding potential}$$

The R0 is the average number of secondary infections caused by a typical infected person in a susceptible population. For example, highly contagious measles has an R0 = 12–18. That means that 1 person can infect about 15 other people and then each of those 15 can infect another 15, and so on. As you can see, measles can spread very quickly. Using a meta-analysis (combined results of many reports), the estimated R0 for COVID-19 is 2.79, meaning that 1 infected person can infect 2 or 3 others.

3

A SHORT HISTORY
OF GERMS

Let's start our story at the beginning. Planet Earth began about 4.5 billion years ago as a hot ball of condensing gas and dust revolving around the sun. The earliest sign of life on earth detectable by science was the germ, also known as the microbe. Fossilized bacterial cells in rocks found in Africa and Western Australia date to 3.5 billion years ago, and the first prototype of cells dates back to about 3.8 to 4 billion years ago. It can be said that germs are indeed the very building blocks of evolution.

Even as the evolution of higher life forms took place, germs never lost their status as the dominant creatures on the planet. The very air we breathe, the water we drink, the food we eat, the ground we walk on, the surfaces we touch—all of it is a teeming, roiling sea of germs. Germs inhabit every inch of our skin, every channel of our bodies. The combined weight of microscopic germs on earth exceeds the combined weight of all living animals and plants. In fact, no living creature could survive for long in an entirely germ-free environment. Without germs, animals, including humans, could not develop mature immune systems or even digest their food (germs break down food in the intestine; they extract and produce essential nutrients and vitamins). The ecosystem of the human body is delicately balanced by germs. Often when we get sick, the problem is that we have disturbed this natural balance and turned our own good and necessary germs against us.

WHAT IS A "GERM"?

The catchall terms *germ* and *microbe* cover a vast array of microscopic forms: bacteria, viruses, fungi, protozoa, and algae. All of their cells are too small to be seen with the naked eye. For example, bacteria are primitive cells with both DNA and RNA. Viruses are even more primitive, containing either RNA or DNA but not both.

WHAT IF THERE WERE NO GERMS?

In order to truly understand the significance and importance of germs to life on earth, let us imagine that there were no germs. Let's say that they died off after higher life-forms had evolved from them. Shortly thereafter, there would be four insurmountable problems on earth: no food, no oxygen, no nitrates, and no recycling of matter and, because of that, **no** life as we know it!

Let's examine these problems one at a time.

NO FOOD: Microscopic cyanobacteria (aka blue-green algae) are the foundation of the entire world's food chain. These lowly germs are eaten by sea creatures and then fish, and then up the chain to land-dwelling animals. If there were no germs in the seas, all marine life would starve to death, and land animals, including humans, would eventually follow suit.

NO OXYGEN: The photosynthesis of land plants can provide only a fraction of the world's oxygen needs. Microscopic cyanobacteria germs supply about 90 percent of the world's oxygen by the process of photosynthesis. This fact highlights the importance of the ozone layer above Earth, because if that ozone layer were to break down and let lethal UV rays hit the surface waters of the oceans, that could also kill the cyanobacteria. Soon thereafter, all the oxygen-dependent species would die of suffocation.

NO NITRATES: Green plants need nitrates in order to grow. And bacterial germs create nitrates by fixing nitrogen, as the process is called. There is a large amount of nitrogen gas that is in Earth's atmosphere, but plants cannot use it directly. In the course of making nutrients for themselves, bacterial germs convert nitrogen gas to nitrates, thus allowing plants to grow.

NO RECYCLING: Organic matter must be decomposed into inorganics in order for the cycles of life to continue. Just imagine generation after generation of plant and animal organisms living and dying, their bodies, their waste matter, and any other organic material they produced piling up on the surface of the earth. Before thousands of years had passed, there wouldn't be an inch of ground left for plants to grow on or for other organisms to live on. The oceans would be thick with corpses. To keep the cycles of life going, nature needs organisms that will break down organic compounds into their fundamental inorganic elements, recycling them for future use. This above all else is the role that germs fill in nature. For every naturally occurring organic compound, there is a species of germ that can break it down and make its inorganic constituent parts reusable. Without germs, all of the earth would soon be one great garbage dump and graveyard, spinning lifelessly in space.

THE NORMAL FLORA

Over eons, germs co-grew with every plant and animal species on earth. In other words, every plant and animal species has its own crew of residential germs, called *normal flora*.

The number of germs in and on the human body actually exceeds the number of body cells by a factor of ten! Over the course of human evolution, many germ species have become beneficial residents in various areas of the human body. They perform life-sustaining tasks such as breaking down food, helping to make essential vitamins and nutrients, and even helping to establish our immunity.

Our normal residential germs—our normal flora—are

located in two major areas of our body. Picture a donut. The outer circle of the donut represents the surface of the skin. The inside of the inner circle represents the respiratory and digestive tracts: the mouth, throat, stomach, intestines, and colon. The area between the two circles represents the internal organs—heart, kidneys, liver, etc.—which are normally germ free. The largest concentration of germs resides in the colon, where feces are formed (that area contains about one trillion bacteria per gram).

Human beings are in a state of dynamic flux with regard to the daily challenges posed by a wide variety of germs in their environment, especially contact with other people. A seesaw relationship exists between humans and germs, whether the germs reside within them or outside them. Most people with healthy immune systems can readily ward off most challenges from *transient germs* (the germs we encounter in the world, some of which may be harmful), although some members of the population—children, pregnant women, the elderly, and the immunosuppressed—will always be at greater risk of infection. Normal flora germs are often closely related, or sometimes identical, to germs that cause disease.

For example, some staphylococci and/or streptococci

can cause boils, abscesses, food poisoning, osteomyelitis, pneumonia, and scarlet fever, among other diseases. And yet there are many different species of streptococci that are common normal, benign flora germs of the mouth (oral cavity). An example can be found in the nose and throat, where *Streptococcus viridans* wards off potentially pneumonia-causing *Streptococcus pneumoniae*. Likewise, *Staphylococcus aureus* and *Staphylococcus epidermidis* are frequently found as normal flora of the skin. Yet if *S. aureus* gets in the wrong place at the right time, it can cause a fatal infection. Some germs do their human hosts a vital favor by actively repelling parasitic germs, or simply by taking up space that the dangerous germ might otherwise invade. Take the bacterial species *Neisseria*, which can stimulate the body to produce an antibody shield against invading meningitis germs (*Neisseria meningitidis*). The skin is a veritable picnic blanket for germs, notably *Staphylococcus epidermidis*, diphtheroid bacilli, and *Proprionibacterium (Cutibacterium) acnes*, and many others are competitive with enemy strains feeding on the oils and dead epithelial cells.

Every germ seeks the ideal environment in which to grow and reproduce. Some of the ecological conditions that affect colonization at a particular site in the human body

include pH (acid/base proportions), moisture, temperature, and other growth factors such as the level of available
nutrients; the presence of supportive or detrimental germs
nearby; and even the influences of magnetic fields. No
single factor will determine the site's suitability, any more
than a house's size alone would determine its attractiveness
to a potential buyer, but a single factor, like the proximity of a house to a noisy freeway, can make a site inhospi-
table to prospective germ residents. Mindlessly responding
to all the ecological conditions involved, germs ceaselessly
seek out and create supportive niches for themselves. In the
process, they gain competitive advantages over other home-
seeking germs. Keep in mind that every area of the donut
provides its own physical-chemical environment, thus allowing for its own particular normal flora residents.

It may be important for us to understand how germs
came to live peacefully in and on the human body. Firstly,
human beings are an excellent host to germs, because they
are a successful species and live a long time compared with
most other animal species. There is a reason why the normal flora germs prefer to live in a mutualistic relationship
as opposed to a parasitic one—if it lives as a parasite, it
might put itself out of house and home by killing the host

too soon. Another important aspect of normal flora germs is that they are protective of the entry points of the body by being competitive with intruding transient germs. I often use the analogy of resident normal flora acting like Roman gatekeepers preventing barbarians from entering the gates of Rome. If there is an intrusion into the body, then our immunity kicks in.

4

HOW WE MAKE EACH OTHER SICK

Scientists call the movement of germs the *chain of infection*. The story of an infectious agent's progress from person to person and population group to population group is called *epidemiology*. Tracking an epidemic literally means tracking what is on people. The first link in the chain of infection is the germ itself, called the *agent*. The agent may be a bacterium, virus, fungus, or protozoon that is found at some source, known as the *reservoir*. We usually associate the term *reservoir* with a body of water, and it could be a body of water, but it could just as easily be an animal or plant that is already home to the germ, or an inanimate object (fomite) that a person has touched.

Some route of *transmission* then transfers the agent to a new *host* organism, completing the chain of transmission (agent–reservoir–transmission–host).

An infectious disease may or may not result at this point. It depends on the virulence of the germ and the health of the host, among other circumstances. Interference or a break in any part of the chain of transmission can prevent the infection. You may also hear medical professionals refer to the *incubation period,* which is the time from first exposure to the germ to the time it takes to manifest symptoms.

There are four possible routes of transmission: *contact (direct and indirect), common vehicle, airborne,* and *vector borne.* Before providing more-detailed information regarding each route of transmission, I'd like to mention that some routes account for more disease spread than others. In fact, direct and indirect contact are involved in transmitting a whopping 80 percent of all infectious disease. That is a profoundly important statement, and I will offer protective responses for contact transmission in the next section (page 37). The other three routes of transmission (airborne, common source, and vector borne) transmit the remaining 20 percent of infectious disease, and I will also provide strategies for their prevention. These four routes are how we make each other sick 100 percent of the time—and this knowledge will empower you to dramatically reduce your chances of getting sick!

CONTACT SPREAD

For contact spread, the prospective host must have actual contact with the source of germs. Contact can be *direct or indirect*.

DIRECT-CONTACT SPREAD involves person-to-person spread. Shaking hands or kissing the face of someone with a cold can easily transmit the cold virus or any other respiratory virus like that causing COVID-19. Coughing, sneezing, or talking in someone's face can transfer germs directly or via aerosol droplets within around 6 feet of the source (some scientists have recorded spread of up to 10 feet). Also, some reports indicate simple breathing can also spread the COVID-19 virus and likely other viruses. Sexually transmitted diseases such as syphilis, gonorrhea, chlamydia, and HIV are also good examples of direct-contact spread (to be abundantly clear, they cannot be spread via shaking hands, coughing, sneezing, or through the air).

INDIRECT-CONTACT SPREAD involves an intermediate object, usually inanimate. Rhinoviruses (cold viruses) and noroviruses (vomit- and/or diarrhea-inducing viruses, aka "stomach flu") can make you sick if you touch a doorknob, phone, computer keyboard, handrail, or other surface that a contagious person has touched recently, and then you touch your eyes, nose, or mouth (or a break in the skin in the case of skin and wound infections), all of which are the conduits of entry into your body.

THE OTHER 20 PERCENT

The remaining 20 percent of infectious diseases that are transferred are *common-source, airborne,* and *vector-borne.*

COMMON-SOURCE TRANSMISSION: Common-source spread involves a contaminated inanimate vehicle (food, water, or other liquid) that serves as a vector for the transmission of the agent to several people.

Common-source spread can become a major news story, such as when packaged food is contaminated with *Salmonella* or *Campylobacter* or a public water supply is contaminated with parasites (like *Cryptosporidium*), all of which can cause vicious bouts of diarrhea and nausea with or without vomiting. Members of at-risk population groups, such as children, the elderly, and the immunosuppressed, may even die as a result of being infected in this way.

Common-source spread of microbes causes some 80 million GI infections each year in the United States. These diarrhea illnesses kill 5,000 to 8,000 people annually. About half of these infections are preventable by practicing good personal hygiene, including good handwashing by all who handle or prepare food.

In most cases, the illness is short-lived and we only treat the symptoms, but some germs require antimicrobial treatment if our normal flora or our immunity cannot contain the infecting germ. Long-lasting symptoms require medical intervention.

AIRBORNE TRANSMISSION: Airborne spread implies the spread of germs over a distance of more than several feet between the source and victim or victims. These germs are in such tiny airborne droplets (less than 5 micrometers) that they don't readily fall to the effects of gravity. The classic example of airborne spread is the transmission of the tuberculosis bacillus (see page 97).

VECTOR-BORNE TRANSMISSION: There are two types of vector-borne spread. One involves the mechanical transfer of germs to a host from the body or appendages of another organism. The second kind occurs when an infected arthropod, like a tick or mosquito, bites another organism (see page 106).

We will discuss these three modes of transmission in Part 2.

PART 2

YOUR EVERYDAY
STRATEGIES

HANDWASHING 101

Before 2020, you probably weren't washing your hands often enough or long enough. Handwashing is the *single* most important thing you can do for your health. Simple soap and water is effective against the COVID-19 virus because the soap disrupts the lipids in the virus. But in general, soap and water is good against any germs because it literally washes them away (see page 47 for how that works).

Wash your hands with soap and water for at least 20 seconds in every one of these scenarios:

- Before eating or drinking
- Before touching your face (especially eyes, nose, and mouth) or a wound anywhere on the body
- After using the bathroom
- If you contaminate your hands with a cough, sneeze, or in any other fashion
- After using a tissue to wipe or blow your nose

- After handling paper money (which generally is dirtier than coins, since metals like copper, zinc, and nickel can inhibit the growth of germs)
- When you enter your home as well as your workplace

Simply put: It is important to avoid touching your face (especially your eyes, nose, or mouth) with hands contaminated on your way to and from anywhere to anywhere.

If soap and water are not readily available, you may use an alcoholic gel of at least 62 percent or more alcohol. Alcohol is not a perfect replacement for soap and water, since it will not kill spore formers like *Clostridium difficile* or noroviruses. To sanitize these, you must wash with soap and water.

KEEP CALM AND WASH YOUR HANDS

Think about this: Every time you suds up with some simple soap and water, you're contributing to the health of the global population. Is there any easier way to do something good for humanity? Here are the four steps for proper handwashing:

1. Wet your hands with warm water and lather with soap.
2. Rub the soapy water all over your hands and fingers, not forgetting to get under your fingernails. Think about buying stiff-bristled brushes for cleaning your nails at home. When no brush is available, scrape your five fingers over the soapy palms of each hand. This drives the soapy water under your fingernails.
3. Do this process for at least 20 to 30 seconds. You should do this to the tune of "Happy Birthday" sung twice consecutively; check the box below for alternative songs with choruses that are 20 to 30 seconds long.
4. If you are in a public bathroom, use a tissue or paper towel to dry after washing and use the towel to close

the faucet if it isn't an automatic-stop faucet. Then dispose of that towel after you open the door outside the bathroom. If there is no waste receptacle nearby, drop that paper on the floor. If enough people do so, there will soon be a receptacle there, as there should be.

BEYOND "HAPPY BIRTHDAY"

Want to preserve the birthday song for your special day? There are plenty of songs with a 20- to 30-second chorus. Just a few include "Truth Hurts" by Lizzo, "My Shot" from *Hamilton,* "Landslide" by Fleetwood Mac, and "Raspberry Beret" by Prince. There are lists online of songs with a 20- to 30-second chorus, and you can simply time some of your favorite songs to find a personalized pick that fits the bill.

WHY SOAP WORKS

In use since ancient times, soap is made by mixing fats and oils with a base. How it works is a more complicated story. Soap contains surfactants. The molecules that make up surfactants have both a water-attracting, or hydrophilic, end, and a water-repelling, or hydrophobic, end. As the soap dissolves in the water, the surfactant molecules lower the surface tension of the water and make it better able to loosen particles on whatever is being cleaned. The surfactant molecules and water then hold the dirty particles in suspension until they are rinsed away. At the same time, soap may kill some microorganisms by disorganizing their component parts.

Temperature is not a critical factor in this process, but if the water is too cold, it will not dissolve the soap as easily, and may be so uncomfortable that you won't wash long enough. It doesn't matter whether you use a liquid or bar soap. Even dish soap works. It's technically a detergent that contains mostly mixtures of surfactants, but it functions in much the same way.

HUMAN INTERACTIONS

You should *always* avoid close contact with overtly sick people. But since it's not always obvious when someone is contagious (including you), you should always take the following precautions.

- Always avoid shaking hands, hugging, or cheek kissing. The flu virus, for example, which spreads more easily than cold viruses, can pass several days before, during, and after symptoms develop.
- Instead, raise your hand and say hi or hello. You could also place your hand over your heart and say hello.
- Cover your cough or sneeze with a paper tissue. Discard the tissue after use and be sure to wash your hands afterward.
- If you don't have a tissue, sneeze or cough into the crux of your arm.
- Don't sneeze or cough into a cloth handkerchief. Handkerchiefs are good for mopping up perspiration, but they become germ reservoirs when we blow our noses and then stuff them in a pocket or purse.

COVER YOUR FACE

The recent COVID-19 virus outbreak brought masks to the forefront of the public consciousness. There are two general types: one is a surgical mask, which is loose fitting, and the other is an N95 mask, a tight-fitting mask that's effective at shielding airborne germs. Unfortunately, a surgical mask is not effective at shielding against airborne particles like viruses, but they are effective when used on people who are already infected in order to prevent or reduce transmission of their germs to others. They may help ease anxiety as well as help keep one's hands from their face.

Surgical masks have a place, especially during an epidemic. Wearing a face covering prevents the spread of virus you may unknowingly have and mollifies a sneeze or cough. During an epidemic, we have to assume that everyone is positive, and so everyone who ventures out should wear a surgical mask. If a surgical mask is unavailable, a homemade mask of cloth (any sturdy cloth will do, perhaps made from an old T-shirt) serves the same purpose—with the added benefit that they are washable. The cloth should be doubled, but any like material can be used.

The N95 should be reserved for medical personnel only, because they are in direct contact with infected people. This is especially important in case of shortages of N95's.

In summary, does a surgical mask completely protect a healthy person from getting a viral infection? *NO.*

Does it prevent the wearer from spouting out a virus, if he or she has it, by coughing, sneezing, talking, or even breathing? *YES.*

And is it a good synergistic companion to social distancing? *YES.*

So wear a mask for other people, just like they're wearing masks for you!

DECONTAMINATING YOUR FACE MASK

Here is a simple method for decontaminating any kind of face mask (including homemade, surgical, and N95 masks): Place the mask in a mesh basket over a source of steam for 5 minutes, then let it air dry. Surgical and cloth masks can be re-steamed until they fall apart, but you can only steam the N95 three times. Of course, you can also machine-wash the cloth masks.

STAYING SAFE IN A PANDEMIC

In an epidemic like influenza, or a pandemic like COVID-19, we may be advised to practice the following additional strategies:

- *Social distancing* requires 6 to 10 feet between people. Other than handwashing, this is one of the most important things that one can do to curb the spread of germs. Some recent studies revealed that sneezes have lingering "gas clouds," including infectious droplets, which remain suspended in air. Another study reported that "microdroplets" from sneezes, coughs, or even by simply talking can remain in ambient air for more than 20 minutes. Even simple breathing has been shown to shed viral particles. This is why it's important to minimize contact with people as well as avoid crowds of people.

- During the COVID-19 pandemic, many people were ordered to *"shelter in place"*; in other words, to stay at home for a period of time. This is a defensive tactic to slow the spread of the germ.

- *Self-quarantine* is different from sheltering in place. Usually applying to a person ill with a contagious infection, it means that you should refrain from contact with any other individuals at all. You usually remain at home or elsewhere for a prescribed period of time (usually 2 weeks or so). To be considered COVID-19 free, the CDC recommends that you need to be free of fever without Tylenol or similar drug and have two consecutive negative viral tests separated by 24 hours.

- *Stay-at-home order* is another option under which people are advised to remain at home or elsewhere until told otherwise. But you may go out to buy food and drugs, or walk your dog, as well as get exercise while maintaining social distancing and wearing a mask.

TOUCH AND GO

It is important to keep the objects you touch throughout the day clean, sanitized, and disinfected, especially objects we bring up to our face, like phones. Cleaning removes debris, sanitizing reduces numbers of germs, and disinfecting kills most everything on a surface. Remember, phones touch tons of surfaces (like tables, counters, desks, etc.) throughout the day, and are touched by our hands, which also touch many other things, so they should be sanitized with wipes, or spray plus paper towels, multiple times throughout the day.

- The number one thing to disinfect multiple times a day is your smartphone.
- Two or three times a day, disinfect anything else that you frequently touch or that is used by multiple people. Over the course of one day, make a list of every item you frequently touch to come up with your own checklist. This list might include:
  - iPads and anything else with a touch screen
  - Water bottle

- Lip balm
- Glasses or sunglasses

- Disinfect daily:
  - Doorknobs
  - Faucets
  - TV controls
  - House phones
  - Computer keyboard and mouse
  - Toys and game consoles
  - Light switches
  - Table tops, hardback chairs, and other surfaces

COMMUTERS BEWARE

Buses, trains, and taxis abound with touched surfaces that act as a collection area and transfer points for germs. After touching these surfaces, do not touch your mouth, eyes, or nose until you have washed your hands or have used hand sanitizer. Keep portable hand sanitizer on you at all times so that you can use it frequently on public transportation and maintain peace of mind.

FIRST CLEAN, THEN DISINFECT

People sometimes use the terms interchangeably, but cleaning and disinfecting are two distinct actions. Cleaning is mechanically removing germs and dirt using soap or detergent with water. While it doesn't necessarily kill germs, it effectively lowers their numbers. Disinfecting, on the other hand, actually kills germs with chemicals. The best practice is to first clean a surface or object with soap or detergent and water to get rid of dirt and grime and as many germs as possible, and then use a disinfecting product to kill the remaining germs.

Just to make things more complicated, we also talk about sanitizing surfaces or objects. This refers more generally to lowering the number of germs, whether by cleaning, disinfecting, or a combination of the two.

Here are your best practices for cleaning and disinfecting objects and surfaces in your home:

- First, clean any visibly dirty surfaces using soap and water or detergent and water.
- Rinse with water.

- Before disinfecting, read the label on the product. Follow the label's instructions about wearing gloves, whether reusable rubber gloves or disposable plastic gloves, and/or eye protection. When using bleach products, for example, always wear gloves.
- Also read the label to find out how long the disinfectant needs to sit on a surface in order to be effective.
- Spray or wipe the surface, and then let the product sit for the required period of time.
- If using a diluted bleach solution, rinse again after waiting five minutes.
- Do not mix cleaners and disinfectants. This can be dangerous.

SPRAY AND WAIT

Most sprays and wipes contain quats (quaternary ammonium compounds), which generally take 10 minutes to work. Some products, however, such as Lysol spray, contain the addition of 58 percent alcohol. Such a product works on two or more time frames. It takes seconds to work on certain germs but minutes on other, heartier germs. For example, it kills most viruses in 10 seconds, bacteria in 5 minutes, and hardy bacteria and hardy viruses in 10 minutes. Simply spray on and let dry without wiping.

Alternatively you can use a disinfectant wipe, like Lysol. The rubbing that wipes require helps to remove more debris and germs. The bottom line? Always read manufacturer's instructions so that you understand the parameters of the disinfectants that you are applying.

KNOW YOUR DISINFECTANT

You might be wondering whether frequent disinfecting may have other adverse health effects. Soap and water is entirely safe. Hydrogen peroxide—the one that comes in a brown bottle—is very safe. It's deactivated by contact with organic compounds (i.e., dirt), so make sure you clean thoroughly before using hydrogen peroxide to disinfect.

Bleach is cheap and very effective. Make sure you wear gloves, and dilute bleach according to the following ratio:

- Add 1.5 ounces, or 3 tablespoons, of bleach to a half quart of cold water.
- Leave bleach solution on surfaces for 5 minutes before rinsing.
- To discard bleach solution, mix it with more water before pouring it down the drain.

The diluted solution lasts for about a day. Take care with metal and painted surfaces, as bleach can be corrosive.

Many products on the market rely on quats, which are safe in low concentrations. The higher the concentration of quats in a product, the faster it can kill germs, and the higher the risk to your health. Other disinfecting ingredients include alcohol, phenol, and chlorine.

The good news is that most common cleaners are effective against the coronavirus; no need to get heavy-duty commercial stuff that can trigger asthma. The Environmental Protection Agency has a list of disinfectants that are effective against the coronavirus: epa.gov/pesticide-registration/list-n-disinfectants-use-against-sars-cov-2.

The bottom line? If you want to keep it safe and simple, soap and water, undiluted hydrogen peroxide, diluted bleach (used with gloves), and 62 percent or higher alcohol concentrations are all great for home use. (COVID-19 virus is killed by as little as 30 percent ethanol alcohol.)

I use a cheap vodka (80 proof; 40 percent ethanaol) as a disinfectant to reduce chemical odors. It's very effective against COVID-19 and is safe for food applications, such as on the skin of soft fruit like bananas, oranges, etc.

WHAT ABOUT VINEGAR?

White vinegar is touted as a safe disinfectant for home use. It does kill some germs when used in its undiluted form, but it's not proven to be effective against the coronavirus.

YOU'VE GOT MAIL

Researchers have reported that COVID-19 can remain on nonporous plastic and stainless steel surfaces up to 3 days, and on cardboard and porous surfaces about 24 hours. The easiest way to decontaminate mail, packages, and boxes is to spray with a disinfectant spray like Lysol or a similar product, which kills most viruses in 10 seconds, most bacteria in 5 minutes, and hardy bacteria and viruses in 10 minutes. Simply spray and let dry without wiping. Alternatively, you can use a disinfectant wipe (like Lysol). Wipes have an added benefit of rubbing, which helps to remove more debris.

One additional method is *delaying* opening mail for a day or two, because the COVID-19 virus does not survive and is not viable on paper for long.

CLEAN YOUR GREENS

When you get back from grocery shopping, make a simple mild solution of bleach: 3 tablespoons of bleach in a half quart of water. Simply dip a sponge in it and wipe every package's surface that is possibly contaminated. Let the solution remain on the surface for 10 minutes before wiping dry.

Another possibility (especially with COVID-19) is to use a soapy solution of water and dish soap to wipe surfaces.

Fruits and veggies can simply be washed in a soapy water solution, then rinsed in water and wiped dry. If a semisolid surface like bananas is suspected of contamination, a cheap vodka (80 proof = 40 percent) can be brushed on before peeling and is very effective.

SHOULD I STAY, OR
SHOULD I GO TO A DOCTOR?

It should go without saying that you should stay home from work or from travel when you are sick with any respiratory infection. Here are some specific scenarios in which you should take extra caution and see a doctor:

- If a cold lasts a week or more without you feeling better.
- If you have a fever (100.4°F or higher) with other symptoms, like cough, shortness of breath, fatigue, flu-like symptoms.
- If you are 65 years old or older, a fever of 99.6°F or higher would be considered a fever, because older people don't usually spike a high fever.
- Severe asthma attacks that do not respond to normal asthma medication.
- Rashes if they look like small bleeding spots beneath the skin, and are accompanied by high fever or sleepiness, or occur inside the eye or mouth.

- A head injury if it causes loss of consciousness, vomiting, sleepiness, difficulty in arousing the victim, change in mental acuity, or headache unrelieved by over-the-counter meds.

- Seizures. Move harmful objects out of the way of the victim, roll onto the left side to prevent choking if vomiting, and start rescue breathing if breathing ceases or is obstructed.

- If there is uncomfortable pressure, fullness, or squeezing pain in the center of the chest lasting two minutes or more, or pain spreads to the neck, arms, shoulders, jaw, or back. These could be symptoms of a heart attack. Take a regular dose of aspirin (325 mg) and get an ambulance.

- If diarrhea and vomiting last more than a day or two (12 hours in the case of an infant) or is severe, or at any time when either is bloody. Most GI bouts are self-limiting and resolve quickly.

- If abdominal pain is accompanied by continual vomiting.

WHEN COWORKERS ARE SICK

If you see a coworker is obviously sick, gently encourage that person to go home and recover for the sake of all concerned. If that person insists on remaining at work, point out any of the disease-spreading behaviors they are engaged in, such as coughing and or sneezing freely without covering, etc. If that doesn't work or if the situation becomes uncomfortable, keep your distance from that individual.

LUNG STORY SHORT

Did you know there's a difference in the quality of air that reaches your lungs depending on whether you breathe in through your nose or your mouth? The nose actually filters and prepares air before it reaches the lungs. When a breath of air enters the nose, it is warmed or cooled to an appropriate temperature, humidified, and then filtered by the small hairs of the nose before moving to the lungs.

Next, the air travels along mucous membranes covered with hair-like cells called cilia, which actually beat and move particle-laden mucus away from the nose. Any impurities are carried toward the back of the throat, where the mucus is swallowed. This defense is called the *mucociliary escalator*. Then the air is ready for the lungs and it moves down the trachea (windpipe). The trachea divides into two bronchial tubes (bronchi). The bronchi further divide into a complex of even finer branches or smaller airways called bronchioles deep inside the lungs.

There are millions of bronchioles in each lung leading to air sacs called alveoli, each of which is surrounded by tiny blood vessels called capillaries. These microscopic alveoli and the capillaries have walls so thin that the delicate membrane allows incoming oxygen to be exchanged for outgoing carbon dioxide. There are about 300 million or so tiny bubble-like alveoli. When oxygen enters the air sacs, it dissolves through the delicate membrane into the blood.

COVID-19 wreaks its havoc by thickening the delicate membranes of the alveoli and capillaries, preventing oxygen from entering the red blood cells. This causes ARDS (acute respiratory distress syndrome) and eventually death by suffocation (hypoxia). Unfortunately, when COVID-19 patients get pneumonia it occurs in both lungs. Fatal cases experience what is called the cytokine storm, which is an immunological overreaction—a systemic inflammatory response syndrome. They also experience cascading multiple organ failure (especially heart and kidney failure). And young and middle-aged people are even more prone to clotting. There may also be an as-yet-unidentified genetic component at play here, especially in fatal cases with younger patients.

WHY DO WE COUGH?

Guarding the air sacs are cells called macrophages. They are a significant line of defense as they trap foreign bodies, including germs, and kill them. Afterward the residue from macrophages works its way to the mucociliary escalator (which extends to the bronchioles) for elimination from the lungs.

Coughing is the body's attempt to clear the airway of excess mucus, dust, debris, or aspirated foodstuff. A chronic cough is a sign of chronic bronchitis, which can have many causes including infection, asthma, tumors, and any airborne irritant.

WHAT IS SHORTNESS OF BREATH?

Shortness of breath (aka dyspnea) is basically difficulty breathing. Sometimes it is described as breathlessness or feeling like you are suffocating. It has many causes besides infection, such as asthma, smoking, allergies, high altitude, obesity, heart or lung disease, and cancer.

STAY SAFE. PERIOD.

Tampons create a unique physical-chemical environment in the vagina, which can turn on toxin production if a woman carries a toxigenic strain of *Staphylococcus aureus* in her vagina and does not have sufficient antibodies for protection. She can get a toxemia, a type of poisoning called toxic shock syndrome (TSS). Symptoms range from a mild, flu-like illness to a severe multisystem disease, often life-threatening. It's characterized by fever of 102°F or higher, a rash resembling sunburn with subsequent peeling of the skin, hypotension, or dizziness. The height of TSS cases was in August 1980 when there were no 100 percent cotton products on the market; since then, most synthetic ingredients have been taken out of tampons. But TSS still occurs; there have also been cases with menstrual cups and cervical caps. Here are some steps for staying safe:

- If you have ever contracted TSS, never use tampons again.
- Leave a tampon in place for no more than 6 to 8 hours.
- Use only the absorbency necessary for your flow.

- Do not sleep with a tampon in; use a pad instead.
- Whenever possible, alternate between the use of tampons and pads.
- Never use a tampon for any reason other than menstruation, unless directed by your doctor.
- Use 100 percent cotton tampons whenever possible, as they provide the lowest risk of contracting TSS.
- If you show symptoms of TSS, remove the tampon and rush to your doctor or ER. Be sure to tell your doctor that you have been using tampons.

PARTY POOPER:
THE FECAL–TO–ORAL ROUTE

The fecal-to-oral route is, unfortunately, exactly what it sounds like: what happens when an infected person fails to practice adequate hygiene after defecating. Feces carry microbes from our large intestine, some of which could be pathogens (i.e., norovirus, hepatitis A, shigella, salmonella). The most common entry point for these types of germs is your mouth. Dependent upon the germ, symptoms vary from periodic diarrhea, abdominal cramping with or without nausea, vomiting, or fever.

This can happen directly—for example, by shaking hands—or indirectly, such as by eating food or drink that was prepared or handled by an unhygienic germ carrier. When you get food poisoning from a salad bar, sandwich counter, or restaurant, fecal-to-oral is usually to blame.

Fecal-to-oral route can also come into play during sexual activity. From kissing to fellatio and cunnilingus, it's easy to see how contamination happens. That said, if neither partner has an STD or other infection, there is no danger of infectious illness from ingesting germs during sexual activity.

If feces contain no infectious illness causing germs, and if you have a healthy immune system, you can literally spoon-eat it without a problem (except, of course, aesthetically).

There's evidence that the COVID-19 virus is present in feces, raising the distinct possibility of fecal-oral transmission. Another study reported that 39 patients were found to be stool positive for from 1 to 12 days. In addition, the stool of 17 of those patients remained positive in their feces even after respiratory samples tested negative. A significant portion of COVID-19 patients experience diarrhea, nausea, and vomiting and/or abdominal discomfort before the onset of respiratory symptoms. Such fecal spread was already found in the 2003 SARS outbreak and is characteristic of some ordinary coronaviruses also.

Of paramount importance is the proper way to wipe one's anus. Consistency of the stool determines the degree of wiping you need to do—the better formed the stool is, the less fecal debris there will be on the anus. To wipe yourself hygienically:

1. Use soft, dry toilet tissue to wipe away as much fecal debris from the anus as possible.

2. Follow with a series of wet tissues using either salt-water or a soap and water solution. In a pinch you can wet tissue with plain water, but plain water should not be routinely used because it may be irritating. Use wet wipes when outside the home. At home, a simple DIY salt solution can do the trick. Simply add a teaspoon of table salt to a glass of water. Continue wiping until there is no obvious soiled toilet tissue. You may alternate between wet and dry wiping for greater effectiveness.

3. Pat dry.

4. Most important, properly wash your hands afterward.

CLEANING AND CARING FOR WOUNDS

Ouch! You might have a simple cut or abrasion, or something a bit more severe like cysts, pustules, boils, or ulcers. However deep the cut or nasty the abrasion, here are some steps to follow:

- Always wash your hands properly (see page 45) before touching any open wound on the body or when you change bandages or dressings.
- Clean the wound with hydrogen peroxide, then disinfect with Bactine, Neosporin, or similar agent.
- Finally, apply a clean dressing to the wound.

WHEN TO SEE A DOCTOR

- If you do touch an open wound with dirty hands, it can result in infections, which are hallmarked by hot, painful, reddened areas (erythema), with hyperemia (swelling), and later weeping lesions oozing pus. See a doctor if this happens.

- A clinician must treat such infections quickly in order to prevent spread and before it becomes a systemic infection.

OTHER TIMES TO SEE A DOCTOR INCLUDE

- If cuts are deep, bleed heavily, cause a loss of movement or function, or have separate edges.
- If burns involve significant blistering or charring, or involve the palms of hands, the soles of feet, the face, or groin.
- If insect bites or stings cause severe swelling, a generalized rash, or difficulty breathing.

KEEPING KIDS SAFE

With their immature immune systems and tendency to put everything in their mouths, children under six are at increased risk of infection from contact spread, as well as other forms of germ transmission. All children need to be taught proper hygiene, and you'll also need to regularly clean toys, objects, and surfaces that young children regularly touch at home. And by all means, children should not attend school or engage in any other activity if they are sick.

To disinfect kids' toys and other objects: Use nontoxic substances like undiluted white vinegar (note that this isn't proven to kill the coronavirus), peroxides, or simple soap and water. There is also a large assortment of child-friendly products available (always read labels; you want to avoid bleach, chlorine, and ammonia). Use a lot of elbow grease when applying these agents.

You might notice a toy—especially a water toy—has become very pungent. This usually means it's really contaminated. In this case, you can use a diluted bleach solution (3 tablespoons of bleach to a half quart of water) to clean that ultra-dirty toy. Then rinse well afterward. Then air dry.

Children also should be taught to do the following:

- To wash hands before eating or drinking, and after using the bathroom.
- To cover their coughs and sneezes.
- To never use someone else's eating or drinking utensils, even if the other person is a relative or their best friend.
- To wash dirty toys after they have been played with on the ground, whether outdoors or indoors.
- To never eat any food that has fallen on the floor or ground. The five-second rule is a myth.
- To wear long pants or skirts when visiting public facilities such as movie theaters, stadiums, etc., where sitting down with bare legs could lead to contracting an infectious illness from germs on the seat.

PAW PATROL

Many germs are transmitted from animals to humans. They're called *zoonotic diseases* and include anthrax, influenza, AIDS, and Ebola, just to name a few—although it's unlikely that your cat or dog is carrying those serious germs. To cohabitate safely with your animal friends, here are a few key action steps:

- Make sure your pets' vaccinations are up to date. Dogs and cats can carry the rabies virus and leptospirosis (caused by a syphilis-like *Leptospira* bacterium), which can be transmitted to human beings.
- Don't let pets stray into the wild. House cats generally are healthier than outdoor cats, who eat birds and mice and thus are more likely to carry *Toxoplasma*, which infects about 2 billion people each year and can cause birth defects. Pregnant women should not clean out a cat's litter box. The *Toxoplasma* parasite can also be transmitted by eating raw or undercooked meats, especially venison, lamb, and pork.

- Wash your hands after cleaning a litter box or using a pooper-scooper. This will safeguard you against both *Toxoplasma* as well as *Toxocara,* a roundworm parasite found in both cats and dogs that migrates in the human body.

- When you stroke or handle your pet, avoid touching your face until you wash your hands. Even a turtle or lizard can carry pathogens like *Salmonella.*

- After kids enjoy a petting zoo, make sure that they wash their hands properly before eating, drinking, or touching their face.

- Keep pets well groomed. A clean, well-brushed dog or cat will suffer fewer fungal infections, fleas, and ticks, and be less likely to pass on these critters to people. Bathe your dog every 2 to 4 weeks; the frequency depends on breed, so make sure you do your research about the specific needs of your dog.

- After giving meds to a sick animal, wash your hands thoroughly so you don't transfer germs to other animals or yourself.

- Keep sick pets isolated from others.

- Don't let a cat or dog get so overexcited while playing

with them that they inadvertently bite or scratch you. In cats this bite or scratch can increase your risk of *Bartonella* infection (a type of cat scratch disease). The bacterium is passed from fleas to cats and other animals and can cause swollen lymph gland disease in human beings.

- Never allow your pets to lick your mouth, nose, or an open wound. Among other germs, they can transmit *Pasteurella,* which could prevent a cut from healing or cause some other type of infection. I have to confess that when my two daughters were growing up, I struggled in vain to convince them to stop smooching their dog. I suppose you could say that when a person and pet have bonded for life, let no man put asunder!

CAN MY PET BECOME INFECTED WITH COVID-19?

Both cats and dogs are found to carry the COVID-19 virus, but thus far neither has been found to transmit it to humans. However, cats were found to transmit the virus to other cats, but not dogs to other dogs. Tigers and minks were also found to have COVID-19 virus, and it is unclear if they can transmit the virus to people. Similar studies were conducted in other animals—namely pigs, chickens, and ducks—and no viral RNA was detected in any virus-inoculated animals or exposed animals.

EATING CLEAN:
HOW TO PREPARE FOOD SAFELY

Remember the fecal-to-oral route? Sorry to bring that up again, but as you may recall, it's why you can get food poisoning when you eat out, and it can also strike at home. Your home kitchen can transmit foodborne germs as well as fecal-to-oral germs—approximately half of foodborne illness can be traced to restaurants and the other half to foods prepared at home—so it's of paramount importance that you practice good food hygiene in the kitchen to keep you and your family safe!

The kitchen almost inescapably contains pathogenic germs from both raw meat and vegetables. In fact, you should assume that the outer surfaces of all fruits and vegetables are contaminated. The number one rule for kitchen safety is—you guessed it—frequent handwashing. But there's lots more you can and should do.

Here are your specific action steps for when you're preparing a meal:

- Wash your hands in between preparing different foods and after completing different stages of preparation. For example, if you've been handling raw ingredients (including vegetables) that will end up being cooked, you don't want to touch another food that will be eaten raw.

- Wash your hands before setting the table.
- This should go without saying, but wash your hands after using the bathroom.
- Also remember to wash your hands after touching inanimate objects such as doorknobs, latches, can openers, countertops, or pieces of furniture while preparing foods.
- Handle food and utensils properly. Be mindful of possible cross-contamination of objects during food prep and the cooking process.
- Cut meats and vegetables with separate knives and cutting boards, or carefully wash knife and cutting board in between the two.
- Fruits and vegetables should be cleaned by soaking for 5 to 10 minutes in a room-temperature solution of water with white vinegar, lemon juice, or vitamin C powder, which you can buy online. Then rinse well to remove any debris. Scald harder raw vegetables like carrots, turnips, and parsnips, or use a veggie brush, which is excellent for cleaning raw vegetables.

- Cook poultry thoroughly. Eighty to one hundred percent of all poultry contains gastroenteritis-causing *Salmonella, Campylobacter,* or both. Never eat poultry if it is pink or bloody inside. Chicken and other poultry should be cooked to an internal temperature of 180°F.
- Cook meat thoroughly. Steak can indeed be cooked rare on the inside, because germs can only reach the outer layer of the meat. Hamburgers, which may contain ground-up bone and other animal parts, should be cooked to an interior temperature of at least 180°F.
- Do not eat unpasteurized cheeses or beverages, such as apple cider. Pasteurization kills diarrhea-causing bacteria like *E. coli* 0157.
- Cook fish thoroughly. Fish can carry the diarrhea-causing germ *Vibrio* as well as parasites.
- Make it a habit never to eat any raw meat, poultry, or fish. And never eat raw eggs unless they are pasteurized. I'm aware many people won't heed this advice; I do hope you don't suffer the possible consequences. And make sure you trust your sushi supplier to be responsible so that you don't get the *Anisakis* parasitic worm.

THE LIFE CYCLE OF LEFTOVERS

Food that's been safely prepared can still become contaminated if served or stored incorrectly. Your instincts have probably kept you away from an egg salad warming in the sun at a summer barbecue—with good reason—but that's just the tip of the iceberg. Read on.

- Don't leave food sitting out at room or outdoor temperature for an extended period of time during cocktail parties, family gatherings, and barbecues. Food should be brought out less than one hour before guests arrive and should be left out no more than two hours in a warm environment. Mayonnaise-laden salads and other creamy foods, for example, provide a hospitable growth environment for *Staphylococcus aureus* germs that are part of many people's normal resident skin flora; this germ can produce toxins in such foods, giving rise to food poisoning in addition to causing infections.
- Also apply the two-hour rule to leftover restaurant food that has been wrapped up to go. Refrigerate restaurant

leftovers as quickly as possible and reheat to 180°F before serving again.

- Reheat and serve leftovers only once, and toss them after three to four days, or when they start to smell off, whichever comes first. Leftover food will have a higher residual bacterial count, and some bacteria (like *Listeria*) can actually grow very well at refrigeration temperature (about 40°F).

- Never store cold cuts and other ready-to-eat foods such as soft cheeses, pâté, coleslaw, and hot dogs for more than a few days to less than a week at most, to prevent the overgrowth of *Listeria monocytogenes*. Pregnant women should avoid such foods.

- Exercise care with the communal plate. During parties, people tend to take second helpings from large serving plates with their own used utensils, which have been contaminated with germs from the skin and mouth (and possibly feces). Or they use their fingers. This is how platters become contaminated, and even worse, bacterial germs can readily multiply. Use separate serving utensils and discourage guests from using their own contaminated utensils.

SUPERMARKET RULES

A simple rule to remember: The older the food, the likelier it is to carry a large quantity of germs. Quantity matters. Ingesting a very large number of some germs will more than likely cause disease even when a smaller amount would have been no trouble at all. Unfortunately, the poor are at greatest risk here. Cut-rate grocery stores often sell packaged foods long past their expiration date, which may have a very high bacterial count. The usual acceptable germ count for hot dogs, for example, is one million per gram, but after expiration may have counts over 330 million per gram. Currently, the legal onus is on the consumer—buyers beware.

Here's what you need to know:

- Always pay attention to expiration dates, and especially check the date on meat, dairy products, and premade salads.
- Ignore the "sell-by" date. That's intended for retailers to know the last day they should keep the product on a shelf. It literally means nothing to consumers. Even

if you buy a product past its sell-by date, it's still likely safe to consume. An expiration date notation like "use by" or "best before" or "best if used by" is the real date that you should pay attention to, indicating when the product is the freshest. No matter what date is printed on the container, if stored properly and left unopened, it is safe to consume long past the expiration date.

- "Organic" does not necessarily mean "safe." Organic produce can harbor pathogens just as easily as conventionally grown foods.
- You may have heard that freezing shellfish for twenty-four hours before eating will kill all pathogens, but that's not true. Cooking is the way to go.

DON'T BE SHELLFISH

Domestic shellfish and bay-caught fish face growing risks of infection from agricultural runoff and from discharge ballast water. Foreign ships typically discharge ballast water into the Chesapeake Bay, a gallon of which contains about three billion bacteria, researchers at the Smithsonian Environmental Research Center found. This discharge includes cholera bacteria, about twenty-five billion virus particles, and unknown quantities of other marine life. Foreign ships empty about 2.5 billion gallons of ballast water into the Chesapeake Bay every year. This additional germ load must be putting great additional stress on the bay and its natural life, which is already under attack from many pollutants, and it could be introducing numerous nonindigenous waterborne diseases into the ecosystem and thus into the food chain. The same thing happens in other bays, harbors, and ports of the American coastlines.

KEEPING YOUR KITCHEN SPOTLESS

It may be hard to believe, but many studies show that the kitchen is actually dirtier than the toilet, with the sink being among the dirtiest areas in the home, especially the drain area. Think about that the next time you place your veggies in the sink for washing! Unless there's something noticeably gross on a toilet seat, it is less contaminated than most people fear. But the kitchen inescapably contains an assortment of potential pathogens from raw meats as well as raw vegetables.

Here's your weekly cleaning checklist:

- Clean the kitchen drain with a mixture of 1½ ounces of bleach in a half quart of water, mixed with liquid soap. Use a brush to clean the drain, since the brush facilitates removal of a biofilm that adheres there. Always wear rubber gloves when using bleach.
- Disinfect clothing soiled while cooking, dish towels, dish rags, sponges, aprons, and linens after each use. They can be cleaned in a washing machine with bleach.

- Spray trash cans with a disinfectant every time you change the bag liner. If you see any liquid at the bottom of the can you must wash it and then sanitize it.
- Disinfect cutting boards with bleach mixture.

POTTY TRAINING

Clean your bathroom weekly—incidentally, that's how often you should clean the other rooms of your home—but there are some special things to keep in mind in the bathroom.

- Carpets and area rugs should not be used in bathrooms, especially in proximity to the toilet. Similarly, don't hang towels or other fabrics near the toilet.
- Always close the lid of the toilet seat before flushing, as small aerosols from the toilet can contaminate surfaces like exposed toothbrushes, faucets, sinks, and counters.
- Because toothbrushes and razors collect cellular debris, they should be rinsed well and air-dried with each use and placed out of range of toilet flushing.
- Don't expect the rim of the mouthwash bottle to be sanitary. Certainly the contents are antiseptic, but there will be a plethora of germs on the spout. It's always best to use a paper cup instead.

- If bath towels are used, they should be completely air dried so that they can be used once more, but should not be used more than twice.

- Clean and disinfect toilet bowls, sinks, bathtubs, and showers (sooner if soiled or dirty) during your weekly clean. Biofilms tend to form on the surface of tubs and only vigorous mechanical action with a brush can eradicate them.

- Loofah and bath sponges capture our skin cells, which serve as foodstuff for germ growth. They should be disinfected weekly with a simple bleach solution (1.5 ounces of bleach in a half quart of water). Wear rubber gloves and, after bleaching, rinse them out with water and set out to air-dry. We shed about 1.5 million skin flakes daily, so it isn't long before they become laden with a variety of germs in the normal skin flora such as *Staphylococcus aureus*, which can cause an infection if it gets into the wrong place.

A NOTE ON PUBLIC RESTROOMS

When you use a public toilet without a lid, be prepared to leave the stall immediately after flushing to avoid the spray of aerosol. That said, unless there is a noticeable liquid or other substance on a public toilet seat, it is less contaminated than most people fear. There is usually a low germ count on the seats—and don't forget you have a skin barrier.

What you should really be worried about is the electric hand dryer. Several research studies show that electric hand dryers found in public bathrooms can spread bacteria into the air and onto your hands. I always carry a paper towel in my pocket to wipe my hands after washing (if one isn't available there), as well as to shut the faucet and to open the exit door.

A LAUNDRY LIST

A few simple steps will ensure that your laundry comes out of the wash as fresh and clean as you want it to be. The goal here is not just to deodorize clothing but to purge all germs.

A note of caution: Several studies reported that a person could theoretically become infected by moving wet clothes from the washer to the dryer, and then touching their eyes, nose, or mouth. So stay mindful of touching your face while you do the wash.

- Don't shake out dirty laundry.
- Always wash underwear separately in hot water (at least 150°F).
- When washing whites, add bleach.
- For non-whites, use a detergent with sanitizing agents (for example, Lysol Laundry Sanitizer); it will work in either hot or cold water. Add this to the rinse load as you would a fabric softener, and make sure you follow the package's instructions.

- Check to see if your washer or dryer has a germicidal cycle. Be sure to use them if possible. This gets hotter than the hot cycle, so be aware that this will be harder on your clothing than a hot cycle.
- Once every other month or so, run an empty cycle with bleach and water to disinfect the washing machine.

UP IN THE AIR

Separate from getting sneezed, breathed, or coughed on, airborne spread refers to the spread of germs over a distance of *more* than several feet.

Germs that spread through the air in this manner must be impervious to the effects of gravity. Airborne infectious organisms are usually contained within droplet nuclei, which are less than 5 microns (five millionths of a meter) or smaller in diameter. Such particles can remain suspended in the air for hours or days, depending upon environmental factors such as humidity and air currents. Airborne should be differentiated from aerosols, which are large droplets greater than 5 microns in size, which do fall to the effects of gravity.

The classic example of airborne spread is transmission of the tuberculosis bacillus. A tuberculosis patient is more likely to spread the disease to other people when confined to a room rather than being outdoors. The enclosed space will allow dangerous concentrations of the TB bacilli to build up as the patient exhales.

Carpets in public places have been found to carry as

much as 200,000 bacteria per square inch, and since they are not often deep cleaned they can be a source of an array of microbes of many types. They can easily be "kicked up" into the air as numerous people walk over them.

WHAT CAN YOU CATCH FROM THE AIR?

The SARS coronavirus of 2003 was an airborne event. Similarly, some researchers have reported that the COVID-19 virus can remain in an aerosol in the air for up to 3 hours, and others have actually reported that it can be spread via airborne transmission. Other examples of true airborne transmission at least in some cases are chickenpox, measles, influenza, smallpox, and *Cryptococcus.*

CLEARING THE AIR

You can't control every environment you pass through, but at least you can keep your home free of airborne bacteria. Here are some ways to clear the air.

- Install a high-quality room air filtration system. Dust carries germs, so you want to filter the air in your home. Introducing some amount of fresh air into the room is also important during the winter, when we tend to stay indoors in airtight rooms. In the summer, keep the windows open.
- Buy an allergy cover for mattresses and pillows.
- Vacuum-clean floors, drapes, and upholstery at least weekly to reduce mites and other allergens. Make sure the vacuum is fitted with air filters to prevent allergens and dirt from being recirculated back into the household air. Central vacuums, which are installed in the building, are particularly good, because they collect debris and vent it at a remote area of the house.
- To kill mites, use the chemical benzyl benzoate, but the dead carcasses can still be allergenic and will need

to be vacuumed up afterward. Steam-cleaning or laundering drapes and upholstery at 131°F or higher will also kill mites, as will dry cleaning.

- Avoid having wall-to-wall carpeting, heavy drapes, and upholstery in your home because they are collectors of dust and allergens. If a rug is needed, area rugs are best because they are easier to clean.

- Respond quickly to any sign of cockroaches or other vermin with appropriate pesticides and traps.

- If you'd like to take more extraordinary preventive measures, explore these options: wearing a respirator or using technology like bipolar ionization (BPI) in HVAC central systems (my preference), UV-C light, HEPA filtration, and other certified systems, which can continuously disinfect the air and kill germs on surfaces in homes and any other buildings and spaces where numerous people frequent.

SWEET DREAMS
OR A NIGHTMARE?

Mattresses and pillows can collect so much debris that they actually increase in weight over time. The debris includes human skin cells, human hair, dust mites, which feed on skin cells and their feces, insect parts, bodily secretions and excretions, animal hair and dander, fungi, fungal spores, bacteria, chemicals, dust, lint, fibers, foodstuff, pollen, soil, sand, cosmetics—you get the point. I did a study with *Dateline* many years ago on older reconditioned mattresses across America. We opened up these mattresses and were shocked to find very heavy quantities of debris. Unless you cover your mattress and pillow with allergy covers, you'll be spending a third of your life on debris, which can exacerbate allergies or asthma.

ROOM SERVICE: YOUR HOTEL ACTION PLAN

A few precautions will guarantee that you'll weather your stay at a hotel unscathed by germs. The safety process starts before you even embark on your travels; when booking a hotel, I always check the reviews for comments about cleanliness and housekeeping.

And then the first thing I do upon entering a hotel room is—surprise!—wash my hands. After all, you likely contaminated your hands on your journey to the hotel. You might have touched money, opened a door, pressed elevator buttons, used handrails, etc.

Next, I inspect the room. For this, I always travel with four items:

- A travel-size disinfectant spray
- Alcohol or sanitizing wipes
- A clear plastic ziptop bag
- A pair of flip-flops.

Here's my inspection and disinfection process upon entering a hotel room:

- Start with the bathroom, which can be a considerable germ hot spot. With a tissue, lift the toilet seat and spray disinfectant on the top and underside of the seat, even if it looks spotless. Let the disinfectant sit according to package instructions before wiping it off.
- Wash glasses or cups with hot soapy water and a hand towel if they are not sealed in a wrapper (I also travel with paper cups, just in case). Apply the same wash technique to the ice bucket if it doesn't have a plastic liner.
- Next, use your wipes on frequently touched surfaces, including faucets, doorknobs, toilet lever, light switches, phone ear and mouthpieces, and clock radio buttons.
- Place the TV remote in a plastic ziptop bag. That way there's no need to sanitize it.
- The bed deserves special inspection. Examine the mattress on at least two sides for bedbugs or their debris. Peel back the fitted sheet and look along the

mattress ribbing for bugs or dried blood stains, tiny white eggs, or bedbug-shed skin (outer shells), which can be transparent or yellowish.

- Also examine the "clean" sheets to be sure they don't look slept in or have any debris.
- If there is a bedspread, it is likely rarely, if ever, washed. Fold it up and place it in a corner of the room with a note advising the housekeeper not to make up the bed with the bedspread during your stay. A duvet tends to be safer, but always protect yourself by keeping the top sheet between you and the duvet. Make sure to fold the sheet over it so that your chin is protected.
- If there are drapes, leave them be. They are usually collectors of debris and allergens.
- Don't walk on carpeting with bare feet. Instead use flip-flops to lessen exposure to fungi and other microbes. Similarly, be fully clothed when sitting on chairs or sofa so as to limit direct skin contact.
- Before taking a shower, squeeze a large dollop of shampoo soap into the tub and let the hot water run for several minutes to decrease the number of germs. Use flip-flops to shower (this is especially important if you have a lesion on your foot).

- I would totally avoid taking a bath. As previously noted, biofilms tend to form on the surface of tubs and only vigorous mechanical action with a brush can eradicate them.

BUG OFF!

Vector-borne spread is the scientific name for transmission of contagions by "vectors"—most commonly, flies, mosquitoes, ticks, and other unfriendly pests. It happens in two different ways. One involves the mechanical transfer of germs to a host (i.e., you) from the body or appendages of another organism. For example, flies with *Shigella* or *Salmonella* on the outside of their bodies can transmit germs simply by alighting on you—or maybe on the juicy apple you're about to bite into. The second kind of spread occurs when an infected animal—usually mosquitoes or ticks—bites you. Rabies, one of the most dreaded vector-borne diseases, is common in skunks, foxes, raccoons, and some species of bats.

Mosquitoes and ticks are the most notorious pests to avoid; here are some steps for steering clear of them.

- Mosquitoes tend to remain very close to where they breed—namely, standing water—so you should eliminate standing water to reduce mosquito breeding. All items that collect water should be drained.

- Spray clothing with DEET to repel ticks. If you are concerned about the toxicity of DEET, there are alternative products like oil of lemon eucalyptus.
- Kill ticks rather than repelling them, by using permethrin. This product should be put on clothing rather than skin and can withstand multiple washes.
- Examine yourself and children carefully for ticks after spending time outdoors. Ticks prefer the warmth of little crevices or bends in the body. Use tweezers to remove ticks (never hands) and try to get it headfirst. If it is deeply attached into the skin, use a hot needle near its rear to loosen it first.
- Keep deer away from your house and garden. The deer population carries the *Ixodes* tick (carrier of Lyme disease bacteria). Some people report success using soap and human male urine; deer don't like the scent of either. But I must report that hungry deer will disregard the aversion to those scents.

MOSQUITOES AND TICKS

Mosquitoes can transmit malaria, yellow fever, dengue, encephalitis, and West Nile fever.

Ticks can transmit Lyme disease, Rocky Mountain spotted fever, encephalitis, rickettsial diseases, relapsing fever, babesiosis, ehrlichiosis, and tick fever.

FLIGHT RISK

Maybe you've racked up a lot of frequent-flier miles and have survived many flights unscathed. And you might conclude that air travel is relatively safe.

Indeed, that assumption is correct. All told, it is estimated that about 2 billion people fly annually, yet only a few significant events are reported. Nevertheless, you may wonder if there is any connection between bouts of a cold or flu and your recent air travel. And what about bouts of dizziness, sore throats, light-headedness, dry or watery eyes, fatigue, hearing loss, difficulty breathing, or anxiety? Can these phenomena also be connected to air travel?

Statistics show that there is a connection between all these conditions and air travel, albeit at a relatively low frequency. A growing number of scientific reports associate an increase in risk for contracting a germ-caused disease, which seems mostly dependent upon the length of your flight.

There have been a number of cases of diseases spreading during air travel over the years. Six passengers contracted tuberculosis on a flight from Chicago to Honolulu, and on a flight from Hong Kong to Beijing, a single passenger coughed continuously. Within eight days, twenty passengers and two flight attendants came down with SARS. Most of the passengers were within five rows of the index passenger.

We know that air travel is probably the chief cause of the global spread of the flu. After the September 11, 2001, terrorist attacks, air travel dropped to the lowest level ever at the time. A Harvard University study showed a direct link between the numbers of people traveling by air and the rate of spread of the flu virus. By restricting air travel, the spread of flu was delayed by two weeks.

In another large study, which involved 155 sick passengers on 146 flights, over 69 different days, influenza and parainfluenza viruses were the most commonly isolated microbes. Using sophisticated molecular methods, the authors of the study identified numerous other respiratory pathogens—namely, adenovirus, coronavirus, respiratory syncytial virus (RSV), *Mycoplasma pneumoniae,* and *Legionella pneumophila.*

Happily, about 80 percent of modern commercial aircraft use vertical airflow and HEPA (high-efficiency particulate air) filters, which should limit passenger exposure to small infectious particles. Planes commonly recirculate about 50 percent of cabin air, after first passing it through HEPA filters. Unfortunately, there is no current regulation that requires carriers to use HEPA filters.

The low humidity of air travel can also increase your susceptibility to a cold, as can the tendency to become fatigued, dehydrated, and anxious. Of course, there is also the fact that people are in close quarters, a so-called closed environment, where shared surfaces can more efficiently spread germs. Traveling can also disrupt sleep patterns, exercise, and eating habits as well as normal handwashing and hygiene practices. The biggest risk of all is that you might be seated in close proximity to a person with overt symptoms.

In the past, when food was routinely served to passengers, food- and waterborne outbreaks had also been periodically reported. Recently there have not been any significant foodborne outbreaks reported, likely because these days few airlines actually serve hot food.

Contaminated water is another issue. Water held in on-flight tanks may be riddled with bacteria, so it's always best to drink bottled water in order to maintain proper hydration. After using the toilet, the task of washing your hands with the dribble of water that emanates from the sink's faucets may be a gamble not worth taking, because that water may likewise be laden with germs. Numerous studies have shown fecal contamination to be present on aircraft sinks, faucets, and door handles. Use an instant alcoholic gel sanitizer or an antibacterial wipe to de-germ your hands after toilet use and also before eating, drinking, or touching your face.

BEFORE YOU FLY

There can be no doubt that the entire process of air travel is stressful. The dehydration, variable air pressure, confinement, crowds, fatigue, poor air quality aboard flights—it can all challenge your immune system. A fully charged immune system is your ally for staying healthy on your adventure.

The day before you fly, make sure to:

- Get plenty of sleep and rest
- Drink plenty of water
- Eat sensibly and take a multivitamin (you'll want to be getting extra doses of vitamins C, E, A, and D_3, as well as B-complex vitamins, which are sufficient in most multivitamins)

And make sure you pack:

- A water bottle that you can fill up after you get through security
- Multiple face masks

- A ziplock bag to place your face mask in when you go through security
- Disinfectant wipes
- Alcohol-based hand sanitizer gel or wipes
- Earplugs
- Sleep mask
- Contact lenses, if you use them (and wear glasses on the flight)
- Any medications you'll need on your trip. Take a few extra days of supply beyond a sufficient quantity, in case you are delayed with your return trip. Be sure to also include your medical devices, such as inhalers, needles and syringes, hearing aids, and other appliances.
- Avoid checking bags so that you can minimize other people touching your stuff and streamline the process of leaving the airport
- Avoid wearing jewelry or anything else that might set off the scanner at security, to avoid further touch points

THE PLANE PROTOCOL

You don't need to resign yourself to getting sick every time you go through TSA. Secure your own mask first and follow these steps to increase your odds of good health during air travel:

- When you get to your seat, wipe down the seat, armrests, and tray with disinfecting wipes. The surfaces on the plane are not frequently disinfected (if ever) and, of course, many people have already touched them before you. Consider your hands contaminated after touching any surface on the plane.
- Sanitize your hands before eating or drinking. Since the water sources on planes are likely contaminated, carry alcoholic gels and wipes with you when you travel. Always sanitize hands before eating or drinking and never put unclean hands in your mouth, eyes, or nose.
- Drink at least eight ounces of fluid (preferably water) for every hour or so of flight. Cabin air is typically extremely dry, with the humidity ranging from 1 to about 15 percent, which can be as bad as or worse than

being in a desert. Staving off dehydration decreases the risk of jet lag and allows for a proper immune response at the body's portals of entry for germs.

- Do not drink alcoholic or caffeinated beverages, as these products can actually contribute to dehydration. Plus, alcohol is an immune suppressant.

- If you are seated close to an individual who is obviously ill, ask to have your seat changed. If not possible, wear an N95 face mask if available; otherwise a surgical face mask will do. In fact, always carry an extra so that you may offer it to the sick individual.

- Stand or move around every two hours, at the very least. Do this because there is some good evidence linking the lack of mobility during a long flight and the development of deep-vein thrombosis (DVT), the formation of blood clots in the legs caused by sitting in cramped conditions for long periods.

- Perform seated exercises every hour. Remove shoes, and do foot exercises like foot flexing, by bending your feet upward, spreading your toes, and holding them for 3 seconds. Next, point your feet downward while curling toes, then hold for 3 seconds. Repeat exercises three times every hour or two.

- Wear glasses, not contacts. Contact lenses dry out in the air onboard and cause irritation and itchy, burning eyes. Pack your contacts and wear glasses instead.

DON'T FORGET YOUR HAND SANITIZER

A recent study reported the presence of MRSA (methicillin-resistant *Staphylococcus aureus*) on 60 percent of aircraft tray tables surveyed and in 100 percent of planes, trains, buses, and subways tested.

SPECIAL CONSIDERATIONS BEFORE YOU FLY

If you suffer from a chronic illness of any kind, consult your physician before flying.

If you're flying with heart disease, diabetes, or epilepsy, wear a MedicAlert bracelet.

Do not fly at all in any of these scenarios: if you've had recent eye surgery; are actively bleeding; are near term pregnancy; have acute gastroenteritis, acute middle ear infection, a bad case of flu, sinusitis, or a cold; have had a heart attack or stroke within the last few weeks; or have a recent head fracture or a tumor. There are numerous other examples of when not to fly; use your judgment!

If you have a chronic respiratory disease or lung condition like COPD (chronic obstructive pulmonary disease) or emphysema, arrange with your airline for supplemental oxygen; security concerns don't allow passengers to carry their own supply. Most individuals on land have oxygen saturation in their blood of about 96 percent capacity, while individuals with a chronic lung disease may have lower levels (around 86 percent). Since most planes fly at about 35,000 feet above sea level, the air contains only about 75 percent of the oxygen that it does at sea level.

BOOST YOUR IMMUNITY

There is growing evidence about the best steps one can take to boost their immunity. There are six primary steps to a healthy immune response and to optimize a longer life span.

Before I share those steps, I want to explain an important factor that also plays a role in longevity: your mother's mitochondria. This may sound surprising, but it's grounded in science. Mitochondria are organelles inside each of our cells, which we believe were derived from bacteria during the evolutionary process. They also have genes that are homologous to bacterial genes. We also know that all of us inherit only our mother's mitochondria. It is from her egg that one can inherit the longevity gene. If there is longevity on your mother's side, you likely will also have the longevity gene. Interestingly, you can't inherit your father's mitochondria because it resides in the sperm tail, which provides the energy for the sperm to travel up the fallopian tubes to fertilize the egg. The tail is then lost when the sperm enters the egg.

Without further ado, here are the six steps to a healthy immune response:

1. **Sleep 6 to 8 hours per night**. During deep sleep (REM), your body works to repair muscles, organs, and many other cell types. Chemicals that actually strengthen your immune system begin to circulate. You spend a fifth of your night's sleep in a deep sleep when you are young and healthy. But that starts to fade over time and after the age of 65, it may drop significantly. Scientists think that REM sleep also helps the brain clear out information that you don't need. The body makes more of some hormones while you sleep and downregulates others. For example, growth hormones go up and cortisol (tied to stress) goes down. Studies show that a good night's sleep has the ability to keep your stem cells, your body's fixers, younger for longer. They repair injuries while our bodies are dormant. You should aim for *6 to 8 hours per night* but no more than 9 and no less than 6 (both are harmful and can cause an increased risk in cardiovascular disease).

2. **Exercise a minimum of 1 hour per day every day.** Yes, every day. Science shows that daily exercise of about one hour, whether it be walking, running, biking, swimming, or the elliptical, is extraordinarily benefi-

cial. Exercise helps decrease the chances of developing heart disease and has been shown to boost immunity. Some studies have shown that even a brisk walk can increase the number of T lymphocytes (T cells, which are an important part of the immune system). Another study reported that exercising up to 60 minutes a day causes immune cells (natural killer cells and macrophages) to come out of their holding sites in the lungs, spleen, and lymph nodes, ready to seek and destroy pathogens. Exercise has also been shown to reduce the release of stress hormones as well as strengthen bones and muscles. Many studies have shown that *all exercise* counts as part of physical activity, whether it be from housekeeping chores, or using stairs rather than escalators, or simply strolling around your neighborhood. And standing is better than sitting, but being a couch potato has the exact opposite effect.

3. **Eat small- to moderate-sized, healthful meals.** Healthful meals should include many vegetables and no processed foods. In addition to eating high-quality foods, consider reducing how much you eat. Experiments were carried out on a variety of animals like fish, mice, and monkeys, and the effect of eating just

above starvation levels was the same—prolongation of life. Of course, no one is expecting you to live at starvation levels, but these studies clearly emphasize that it is *not only what you eat* but also the *quantity of food you eat.* A major study published in 2015 reported that people with calorie restrictions saw an increase in many positive indicators of health. In short, calorie restrictions may be one of the most promising avenues for improving both health and longevity.

Returning to the question of *what* to eat, the Mediterranean diet has been shown to be beneficial. As for specific supplements for boosting immunity like vitamins D_3, A, C, and minerals like zinc and magnesium, there's no need for megavitamins. Most available OTC multivitamins are sufficient as daily supplements. Just be sure you are not deficient.

4. **Reduce stress.** Of course, this isn't easy. Most people are aware that stress can be a killer. Stress also plays a role in colds and flus, and for most people summer is a less stressful time than winter. The shorter, darker days of winter also add stress to a large group of people who suffer from SAD (seasonal affective disorder). In one study, 55 volunteers suffering with SAD were

infected with a cold or flu virus, after being interviewed beforehand to determine their psychological stress level. Researchers found that those with high stress levels suffered more severe respiratory symptoms, greater mucus production, and higher levels of interleukin-6, a protein that stimulates inflammatory and autoimmune processes. This study, among many others, implies that stress can intensify cold and flu symptoms, thereby affecting immunity. Be aware of the effects of stress and learn healthy ways to manage it. You can explore mindfulness and meditation as useful tools for stress management.

5. **Be optimistic.** Individuals who are moderately aggressive or assertive personality types are less susceptible to getting sick in the first place. If you are not naturally assertive, a positive attitude of optimism will go a long way.

6. **Practice good personal, food, and household hygiene**, the tenets of which have been delineated within the pages of this book. I hope that, by becoming familiar with its content, you'll be better able to understand as well as block the chain of transmission of infectious diseases, which is still a major

killer worldwide—in fact, it's the number one killer of people in third world countries. Industrialized nations have supposedly relegated germ-caused death to third place after heart disease and cancer; however, because new research implicates germs in a substantial proportion of cardiovascular diseases and cancers, we may once again have to recognize infectious diseases as the worst killer of humans, even in industrialized nations.

With improved awareness of hygiene, many lives can be saved around the world.

PARTING WORDS

No one can avoid all risk. It's a part of life. However, you can keep calm and minimize many risks once you're empowered with knowledge. Your health depends on everyone's sense of responsibility and concern for one another—we are all connected. The flip side of that, though, is pretty inspiring. While you can't save the whole world at once, you can improve the world's health one person, and one person-to-person interaction, at a time.

In short, the first step to improving the health of the planet is to take care of yourself. That will go a very long way in keeping yourself safe, too. Don't panic, wear a face mask, wash your hands, and you'll already be making a difference.

ACKNOWLEDGMENTS

Writing a book during a raging pandemic, the worst of my lifetime, is an experience that is filled with mixed feelings. On one hand I felt some comfort in that I was providing helpful information in the form of protective response strategies for infectious diseases, while on the other hand witnessing the extraordinary incidence of death and suffering caused by the COVID-19 virus was sad and sobering. Nevertheless, the experience proved to me that science prevails because it provides the framework to extricate humanity from the horrors of germ events, but only if we all heed the knowledge gained over the past two millennia. Unfortunately, as the cartoon character Pogo once uttered, "We have met the enemy, and he is us."

While writing this book, I have had the benefit of working

with a skilled senior editor, Donna Loffredo of Penguin Random House. I thank her for her insightful editing and for enthusiastically guiding the book to completion. I also thank her colleagues for their assistance, especially editorial assistant Katherine Leak.

I am grateful to my wife, Josephine, who had to listen to many iterations of various sections of the book ad nauseam. I thank her for her patience and for being my best sounding board.

INDEX

ABOUT THE AUTHOR

Dr. Philip M. Tierno, Jr., is a microbiologist with more than forty years of experience in the field of Clinical and Medical Microbiology. He was the Director of Clinical Microbiology and Diagnostic Immunology at Tisch Hospital, New York University Langone Medical Center, and is currently Professor of Microbiology and Pathology at the New York University School of Medicine. Dr. Tierno has been recognized extensively for his numerous contributions to the medical and scientific community, including the honor of Knighthood by the Sovereign Military and Hospitaller Order of St. John of Jerusalem of Rhodes and of Malta for his work on toxic shock syndrome. His work has appeared in publications such as the *American Journal of Public Health*, *Journal of Clinical Microbiology*, *JAMA*, and *Journal of Infectious Diseases*, and he is the author of several books, including *The Secret Life of Germs*, *Protect Yourself Against Bioterrorism*, and *Nuclear, Chemical and Biological Terrorism: Emergency Response and Public Protection*. He has appeared on both local network and cable television shows, including *20/20*, *Dr. Oz*, *Good Morning America*, *Oprah*, *The Montel Williams Show*, *Dateline*, *Nightline*, *Today*, *Primetime*, *Katie*, *Cuomo Prime Time*, and CNN.